Treating At Home

Remedies for Common Ailments

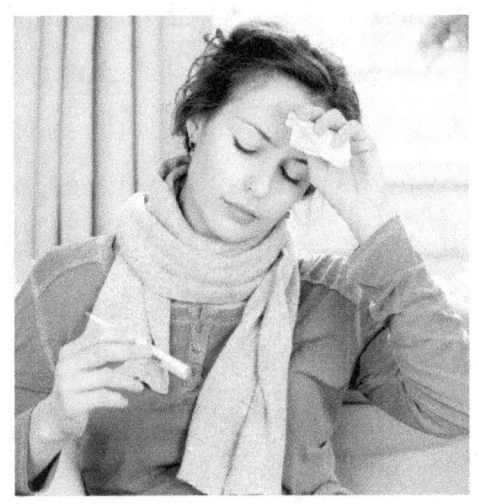

By

Paolo Jose de Luna

Paolo Jose De Luna

This document is geared towards providing exact and reliable information in regards to the topic and issue covered. The publication is sold with the idea that the publisher is not required to render accounting, officially permitted, or otherwise, qualified services. If advice is necessary, legal or professional, a practiced individual in the profession should be ordered.

The information provided herein is stated to be truthful and consistent, in that any liability, in terms of inattention or otherwise, by any usage or abuse of any policies, processes, or directions contained within is the solitary and utter responsibility of the recipient reader. Under no circumstances will any legal responsibility or blame be held against the publisher for any reparation, damages, or monetary loss due to the information herein, either directly or indirectly.

Respective authors own all copyrights not held by the publisher.

The information herein is offered for informational purposes solely, and is universal as so. The presentation of the information is without contract or any type of guarantee assurance.

The trademarks that are used are without any consent, and the publication of the trademark is without permission or backing by the trademark owner. All

Paolo Jose De Luna

Table of Contents

Treating At Home

INTRODUCTION

Nowadays, it is almost not safe to just go wander about everywhere. That includes in the comfort of your own home. It is almost hard to believe that the most common household ailments can also be the deadliest and the most contagious kind of disease.

For starters, these common ailments are merciless, and don't discriminate. They can strike at almost everywhere and anyone. No one is safe against these common ailments. From children to adults, everyone should be careful and be mindful when one strikes. Of course, it's hard when one of our beloved family members gets infected, but that doesn't mean it can't be stopped.

It is equally important for everyone to be always clean and healthy to combat and prevent these common ailments so it doesn't get to the point where one needs to be brought to the hospital.

So just what are these common household ailments? And what do we do to prevent and possibly find a remedy for them? Well, this book will give you an answer to all your questions.

This book will help you understand each health condition and their recommended treatments. You will also learn some of the best remedies that can help you preventing them.

What Are Common Ailments?

Common ailments are some disease, sometimes viruses that have a very high prevalence rate. In other words, these ailments can infect almost anyone from children, adults and elders alike at anywhere from schools, parks, workplaces and even your home. Most people see that common ailments are almost harmless at first, but what some people forget to understand is that these common ailments can turn deadly and take things for the worse when not prevented and treated immediately. Fortunately, these common ailments have simple cures and medicines readily available almost in any pharmacy, making them easy to prevent and then treat later on. These common ailments can take on many forms from simple body aches or colds.

When not treated early, these common ailments can give way to even more lethal disease and may probably result in death. When you think that you may be suffering from these kinds of ailments, it is important to get them treated right away. See a doctor immediately when you feel like you're suffering from any kind of these common ailments to know what it is you are really suffering from so that you may know what

Treating At Home

kind of treatment you can do to get
it treated.

Common Household Ailments

There are many common ailments that can strike at any moment anywhere. Out of all the common ailments that we know today, these ailments are the ones that stand out the most. These are just a few of most ailments:

Common Colds

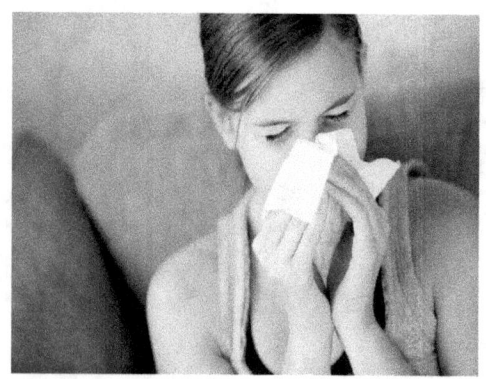

Treating At Home

A common cold is a kind of illness that primarily affects the nose. This is caused by a viral infectious disease through upper respiratory tract. While there is no known cure for common colds, it can be prevented on its early stages. Common cold has been one of the most contagious diseases to humans since ancient times. An average adult would get about two to three colds a year while children can get six to twelve. Signs and symptoms for common colds usually include a runny nose, nasal congestion, sneezing, sore throat, and coughing. If not prevented and treated immediately, common colds can regress to fever or flu over time and can be difficult to prevent.

Treatment for Common Colds

While there is no known way to cure common colds, there are still plenty of ways to prevent it from spreading to the entire household and lessen its effects. A way to reduce the risk of spreading the virus that causes colds is through physical means. These include from daily hand washing ad through wearing face masks. In some cases, vaccination of cold viruses has proved to be difficult as there are so many viruses involved and they mutate rapidly. This fact makes the creation of an effective   vaccine   highly improbable.

Home treatment isn't anything new for common colds. Hydration is one of the most important things that you can do, along with eating more fruits and vegetables since they serve as natural antibiotics. Bed rest is also important to allow the body to relax and recover.

Honey and ginger juice is one of the most effective natural and home remedies for cough. Ginger eases the cough while honey serves as a soothing liquid to the throat and also lessening the pungent smell and taste of the ginger. All you have to do is take

100 grams of ginger, grinding them to paste and then mixing it in a solution of honey and water. The minimum dose of honey and ginger juice is about one teaspoon, but you can take as eight teaspoons in a day.

Headaches/Migraines

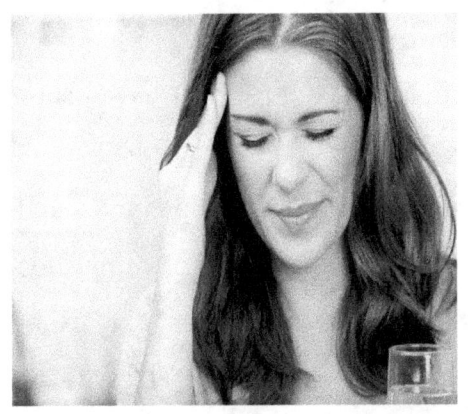

Anyone knows what a headache means. Headaches are pains which originate near the head area usually around the cranium, the face or the neck. Headaches have many causes. Because of the many causes of headaches, it is classified as either primary or secondary. Primary headaches mostly occur on people around 20 to 40 years old. The most common primary headache is migraine. Migraine is a kind of neurological disease and pain is described to have a pulsating sensation. Migraines usually last at around 2 to 72 hours. The headache usually affects one side of the head. Secondary headaches are usually caused by problems elsewhere in the head or the neck. Some of these headaches are not harmful.

Treatment for Headaches/Migraines

Treatment for headaches completely depends on its underlying cause, but mainly involves the use of some pain killers. Some forms of headaches usually give the person a great sense of discomfort.

Migraine can be somewhat improved through lifestyle changes, but most people require medicine to control their symptoms. Medications are either to prevent migraines or reduce its symptoms once migraine starts. These preventive medications are usually required when people have more than four migraine attacks per month, the headaches last longer than 12 hours or the headaches are very disabling.

One effective home treatment for headaches is by using essential oils made from peppermint and lavender. All you need to do is apply it to your temples and you can soothe the headache. Aside from headaches, lavender and peppermint oils can also help in relieving allergies, stomach pain, and joint pain. Massaging the temples can also help ease the pain in headaches, but resting is of utmost importance to limit the stress that the body endures during this time.

Skin Rashes and Irritation

Most skin rashes are caused by irritants mostly located around the environment. These irritants range from chemicals, heat or even some common household pests like flies and mosquitoes. Common skin rashes are prickly heat or allergies either from cosmetic products or any cleaning agents. Skin irritation is one of the most problematic common ailments. Skin irritation can cause itching, inflammation and sometimes even scarring and sores.

As for home treatment of rashes and skin irritation, there are a lot of things that you can use. One of the most well-known home remedies is apple cider vinegar which is a great organic and natural anti-septic and anti-fungal that you only need to apply a small amount on the affected area using a cotton ball. Other home treatments also include oatmeal, peppermint, and aloe Vera as they help relieve the skin of irritation and itchiness.

Allergies

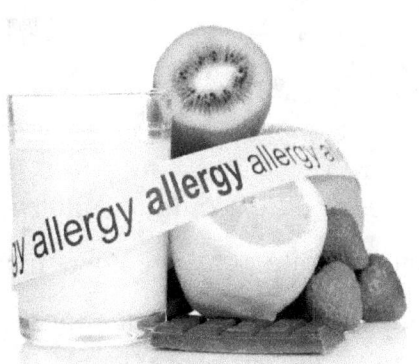

Allergies are a number of conditions caused by hypersensitivity in the immune system to something in the environment which initially causes little problems at first. These include food allergies, dermatitis, asthma and possibly anaphylaxis. There are many varying symptoms for allergies which include skin rashes, red eyes, runny nose, swelling and sudden shortness of breath or hyperventilation. Cases of food poisoning and food intolerances are separate conditions.

Some of the common allergens include pollen or food. Food, insect stings and some medications can also cause severe allergic reactions Metals and other substances may also cause problems. Identifying allergy is almost based on the person's medical history. The cause of allergies in the first place involves around immunoglobulin E antibodies (IgE), which are part of the body's immune systems, which binds to an allergen and triggers the discharge of released elements such as histamine. Early exposure to any potential allergies may also be productive.

There are some forms of allergies that can initiate a severe reaction called "Anaphylaxis". Anaphylaxis is a life-threatening condition and can cause a person to go into shock. The symptoms for this condition include loss of consciousness, drop in blood pressure, shortness of breath, skin rashes, lightheadedness, rapid or weak pulse, possible nausea and vomiting.

Treatment for Allergies

Treatment for allergies completely depends on its root cause. These involves avoiding what triggers the allergy and by using medication to lessen and improve its symptoms. Allergen immunotherapy may also be useful in preventing these allergies.

Several medications maybe used to block the action of allergic mediators which cause the allergic reaction or to prevent activation of cells and degranulation processes which can trigger an allergy. These include the use of glucocorticoids, epinephrine, anti-histamines, theophylline and cromolyn sodium. Anti-leukotriene agents like montelukast and zafirlukast, are treatments of allergic diseases. Drugs like decongestants, anticholinergic drugs, mast cell stabilizers, and other compounds are thought to impair eosinophil chemotaxis which can aid in relieving allergies. Epinephrine has an important role in anaphylaxis as it can lead to the matter of life or death in emergency cases.

Allergen immunotherapy is useful for environmental allergies, insect bite allergies, and also asthma which involve exposing people to bigger amounts of allergen in an effort to alter the immune system's response. Eucalyptus oil can also help control allergies by killing off dust mites, a common cause of allergies, if you wash clothes and bed sheets in the said oil.

Hiccups

A hiccup is a form of involuntary action or jerking of the diaphragm that may repeat for several hours or minutes. The possible cause of hiccups is most likely a misfired message from your brain that gets stuck on an infinite loop. While they're not actually life-threatening or any danger to health, hiccups can get very annoying and problematic when not treated immediately. Hiccups may occur individually or in bouts. In fact, the rhythm of hiccups tends to be consistent.

A bout of hiccups, in general, resolves itself without any

intervention, while some recommend some home remedies to lessen the duration. For chronic hiccups, medical treatment is occasionally necessary. In some clinical cases, it mentions that the lesions of the medulla that involve the area are slightly vertebral and lateral to nucleus and tractus solitarus cause hiccups.

One of the several explanations for this result is that such a lesion "aggravates" descending information from the nucleus solitaries to the phrenic nucleus. It's made up of related groups of cell bodies in the vetral horn from C3-C5. Axons arising from the phreni nucleus comprise the phrenic nerve, which then innervates the diaphragm. This, hiccups result from spasmodic lowering of the diaphragm that causes a short, sharp cough. Brain stem lesions concerning the area ventral and lateral to nucleus and tratus solitaries result in hiccup.

Treatments for Hiccups

In general, a bout of hiccups usually resolves itself without any form of intervention whatsoever. Although, there are still many today who still rely the use of home remedies in an attempt to lessen its duration. Medical treatment is occasionally necessary in cases of chronic hiccups.

There are many superstitious and folk remedies for hiccups, including head standing, drinking a glass of water upside down, having someone surprise you, breathing into a paper bag, and eating a spoonful of peanut butter. Even putting sugar on the tongue has also been used.

A simple treatment for hiccups usually involves by increasing the partial pressure of Carbon Dioxide, and then inhibiting diaphragm activity by holding one's breath or re-breathing back and forth into a paper bag. Stimulating the vagus nerve is also reported to have helped. This can be done at home by irritating the pharynx by either swallowing dry bread or crushed ice, applying some traction to the tongue or by simulating a gag reflex.

Body Pains

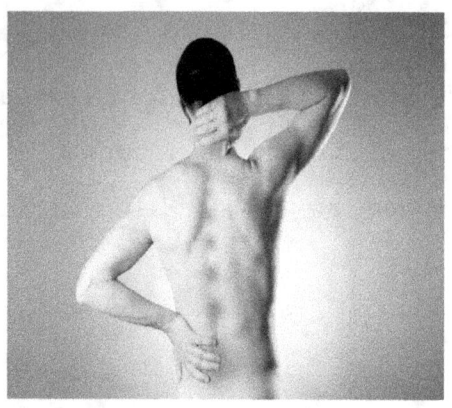

No matter what your age is, no one is exempted and bound to experience body pains which may include headaches, abdominal cramps, joint pain, back pain and a lot more. Body pains have different causes. These range from stress, strenuous activities, sitting or standing for a long period of time, too much physical activities, and even eating something bad. It is always important to be aware of what kind of body pain or for constant your body pain is. For all anyone could know, it may be a symptom for another type of ailment. The most obvious symptom for are muscle or joint pains.

Treatments for Body Pains

There are plenty of ways to prevent some common pains. These are either through physical means, lifestyle means or the use of medication. For muscle pains, many usually recommend prevention through the use of indirect ice. Applying ice in some parts of your body with muscle pains won't actually prevent muscle pains, but it can lessen the effects. This same principle also works with back pains and possibly some joint pains. If you get sore muscles often, you can also take acetaminophen or a nonsteroidal anti-inflammatory drug (NSAID) like aspirin, ibuprofen, or naproxen to help ease the discomfort. For abdominal pain, using home remedies like fennel, ginger, and tea can help in limiting abdominal cramping which ease the pain.

Acne

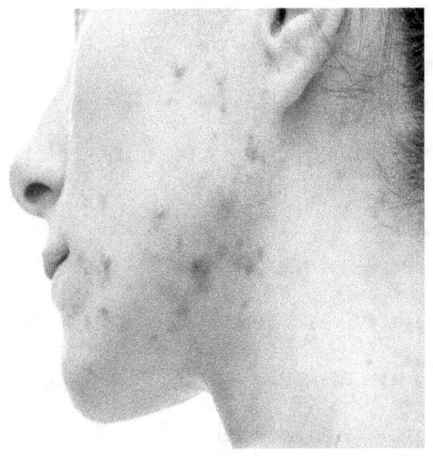

Simply known as acne, Acne vulgaris is a long-term skin condition which is characterized by blackheads, whiteheads, pimples, greasy skin and possible scarring in the affected areas. For one who is suffering from this condition, they may experience anxiety, depression, low-self-esteem, and at worst, even self-harm or suicide. In studies, it is thought that the 80% cause of this condition is through Genetics. The cause is also unclear for the role of diet. Cleanliness or sunlight is not involved in the cause of acne. It is shown that cigarette smoking also increases the development of acne and can also make it worse. Acne mostly affects the skin mostly with the greater number of oil glands including the face, upper part of the chest, and at the back. Acne is often brought on by an increase in androgens like testosterone during puberty in both genders. Too much growth of the bacteria *Propionibacterium acnes*, which is most of the time found on the skin.

Treating At Home

Acne mostly occurs during adolescence, affecting over 80% to 90% of teenagers in the world. Lower rates of acne are also reported in rural areas, most probably because of lesser pollution. Acne affects usually around 650 million people globally, making it as the 8th most common disease worldwide. Acne can also occur even before or after puberty. While it is less common in adulthood than in adolescence, almost half of people in their twenties and thirties still experience acne. About 4% of people worldwide still experience acne even in their forties.

The severity of acne is often divided into three classifications – mild, moderate, or severe. Mild acne is commonly defined as open and closed comedones limited to the face with sporadic inflammatory lesions. Those with a higher number inflammatory papules and pustules occur on the face are considered to be of moderate severity, and some acne lesions may also occur on the trunk of the body. And lastly, severe acne is said to occur when lumps and cysts are the characteristic facial lesions and involvement of the trunk is extensive.

Treating At Home

While the connection between acne and stress is still unclear, some studies have shown that increased acne development may be associated with high stress levels. One type of acne, acne excorie, occurs when a person picks and scratches pimples due to stress.

Scars caused by acne result in inflammation within the dermal layer of skin brought about by acne and are likely to affect 95% of people with acne vulgaris. Scars are created through an abnormal form of healing following this dermal swelling. Scarring is most likely to happen with severe nodulocystic acne, but it can also occur in any type of acne vulgaris. Acne scars can be classified based on whether the abnormal healing response following the dermal inflammation leads to excess collagen deposition or collagen loss at the location of the acne lesion.

One of the most common types of acne scar like Atropic acne scars has lost collagen from healing response. Atropic scars may be further classified as ice-pick scars, boxcar scars, and rolling scars. Ice pick scars typically look like narrow, deep scars that extend to the dermis. Rolling scars are wider than ice pick scars and follow a wave-like pattern of depth in the skin. Boxcar scars are round or avoid any indented scars with sharp borders and vary in size from 1.5 to 4 mm across. Hypertropic scars are not so common and are characterized by increased collagen content after the abnormal healing response. Hypertrophic scars remain within the original margins of the wound, while keloid scars can form some scar tissues outside the borders. Hypertrophic scars are described to be as firm and raised from the skin. Keloid scars from acne usually occur on men and form around the trunk of the body rather than the face.

Treatment for Acne

Usually, the result of nodular or cystic acne is post inflammatory pigmentation (PIH). They often leave behind some inflamed red marks after the original acne lesion has resolved. PIH occurs more on people with a darker skin tone. While pigmented scarring is common, it is a misleading term since it suggests that the color change is permanent. PIH can be avoided by avoiding any aggravation of the nodule or cyst or by refraining from touching, scratching, or popping the acne. These scars can fade over time. Some untreated scars however, can last for months, years or may even become permanent if deeper layers of skin are affected. Daily use of sunscreen or SPF 15 can help minimize the pigmentation associated with acne. If you want a more natural approach to treating acne, eating more cherries and other berries may help since they are considered to be organic anti-inflammatories.

Diarrhea

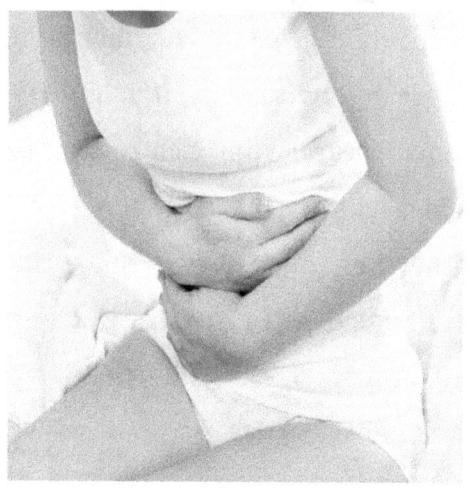

Diarrhea or loose bowel movement is a condition in which a person experiences having at least three loose or liquid vowel movements each day. This sometimes lasts for a few days and can result in dehydration due to loss in fluids. Sins of dehydration may begin with loss of the normal stretchiness of the skin and changes in personality. This progresses further to loss of skin color, faster heart rate, decrease in responsiveness and decreased urination as it becomes more severe.

The most common cause of diarrhea is through an infection of the intestines either due to a virus, bacteria or a parasite. This condition is also known as gastroenteritis or AGE. This type of infection is every so often acquired from food or water that has been contaminated by stool, or straight from another infected person.

The extent of severity caused by diarrhea may be divided into three types: short duration ad watery diarrhea, short duration and bloody diarrhea and if it lasts for more than 2 weeks, it is persistent diarrhea. Short diarrhea is usually due to cholera. If blood is present, it is a case of dysentery. A number of non-infectious causes may also lead to diarrhea like irritable bowel syndrome, lactose intolerance, hyperthyroidism, inflammatory bowel disease and a number of medications.

About 1.7 to 5 billion people get infected of diarrhea per year. It is one of the most common diseases in most developing countries, where young children mostly get diarrhea three times a year.

Diarrhea is also one of the most leading causes of deaths in children where it ranked at second in 2012. Total deaths from diarrhea have an estimated figure of 2.58 million between 1990 and 2013. Frequent episodes of diarrhea is also a common cause for malnutrition and one of the most common cause in children from five years of age or may even be younger like infants and toddlers. Other long term complications of diarrhea in children may include dehydration, stunted growth, and intellectual problems.

Paolo Jose De Luna

Treatment for Diarrhea

Prevention of diarrhea can be improved through proper hygiene and strict hand washing with soap. For mothers, breastfeeding for at least six months is much recommended as is a vaccination against rotavirus. One of the recommended treatment choices is through oral rehydration solution, through the use of clean water with modest amounts of salts and sugar. Zinc tablets are also recommended. For people who have diarrhea, it is recommended that they have a balanced diet and eat healthy food, and babies continue to breastfeed. If any commercial ORS are not available in one's locale, some homemade solutions may be used. Some intravenous fluids may be required for those with severe dehydration. While rarely used, antibiotics may also be recommended in few cases such as those with bloody diarrhea and high fever, those with severe traveler's diarrhea and those who cultivate specific bacteria or parasites in their stool. Loperamide may also help decrease the number of bowel movement but is not recommended in people with severe diarrhea. Probiotics (gut-friendly bacteria) from yogurt and other fermented foods can also help promote healthy intestinal flora.

Constipation

Constipation, costiveness, or dyschezia is a condition refers to bowel movements that are infrequent or hard to pass out. Constipation is one of the most common causes of painful defecation or passing out of stool. Severe constipation fecal impaction, which can further progress to intestinal obstruction if not treated accordingly and may become life-threatening.

There are many causes for constipation. There are usually two types: obstructed defecation and colonic slow transit. Between the two, obstructed defecation is the most common. This type of constipation has mechanical and functional causes. The causes of the slowing of the colonic movement include diet, hormonal disorders like hypothyroidism, side effects through medication and rarely heavy metal toxicity. Because of the fact that constipation is a symptom and not a disease, determining the cause of constipation is essential before starting the treatment

The causes of constipation can be divided into either congenital, primary or secondary. Primary is the most common cause of constipation, but is not life threatening. In older people, causes of constipation may include insufficient dietary fiber intake, impaired physical activity, not drinking enough water, side effects from medication, hypothyroidism, and obstruction by colorectal cancer. Constipations with no known cause exhibits gender differences in prevalence: females are usually more affected than males.

Primary or functional constipation is continuing symptoms for more than six months not due to any underlying cause such as medication side effects or any underlying medical condition. This is not particularly associated with abdominal cramping or pain, thus it can be ruled out from irritable bowel syndrome, a common cause of constipation.

Constipation can also be caused by an exacerbation of a low-fiber diet, low liquid intake or dieting.

Any metabolic and endocrine problems may also lead to constipation. These problems include: hypothyroidism, diabetes mellitus, cystic fibrosis, hypercalcemia and celiac disease. Constipation may also become common in individuals with some muscular and myotonic dystrophy.

Constipation has many structural causes. These include spinal cord lesions, Parkinson's disease, anal fissures, colon cancer, and pelvic floor dysfunction. Constipation also has functional causes, which include: anismus, descending perineum syndrome and Hirschsprung's disease. Among infants, this is the most common medical condition associated with constipation. Anismus occurs in small minority of people with chronic constipation or obstructed defecation.

A common cause of constipation is voluntarily withholding stool. This choice may be brought about through psychological means like fear of pain, laziness or fear of public restrooms.

Treatment for Constipation

Treating constipation include applying changes in the diet particularly eating food rich in fiber, use of laxatives and enemas, exercise, and biofeedback or in some particular cases, surgery may be required.

There are many medications that have constipation as a side effect. Some of these include opioids (also known as narcotic drugs), diuretics, antidepressants, antihistamines, anti-spasmodic drugs, anticonvulsants and some aluminum antacids.

Fever

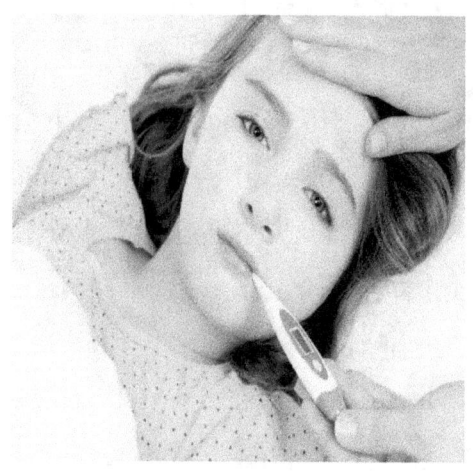

Also known as pyrexia and febrile response, fever is defined as having a temperature that is above the normal range due to an increase in one's body temperature set-point. This increase in body temperature in set-point triggers increased muscle contraction, and causes a feeling of cold. This results in higher heat production and efforts to conserve heat. When the condition subsides, the person may feel hot, becomes flushed and begin to sweat. Almost rarely, a severe fever may also trigger a febrile seizure which is more common among children. Fevers do not typically go higher than 41 to 42 °C (105.8 to 107.6 °F), but at this level, it is already considered as dangerously high.

A fever can be caused by several medical conditions which range from not serious to potentially serious. These conditions include viral, bacterial and parasitic infections like common colds, urinary tract infections, meningitis, malaria and appendicitis. Non-infectious causes include vasculitis, cancer, deep vein thrombosis, and side effects of medications among others. Fever is different from hyperthermia; in that hyperthermia is a rise in body temperature over a set-point due to either too much heat production or not enough heat loss.

Fever is said to be one of the most common medical signs. It is a part of almost 30% of healthcare visits by children, and has at least a 75% chance to occur among adults who are seriously sick. While it can also be a useful defense mechanism of sorts, treating fever does not seem to worsen some outcomes. Fever is viewed with greater concern by both parents and healthcare professionals than it usually deserves, a phenomenon known as "fever phobia".

Treatment for Fever

Treatment to resolve a fever is often not required. Most often, treatment only includes bed rest for a couple of hours or even a day. This is because most people usually recover without requiring any specific medication attention. It may be unpleasant to some, but fever rarely rises to a dangerous level even if untreated. Any damage to the brain does not occur until temperatures reach 42 °C (107.6 °F). It is also rare for an untreated fever to grow more than 40.6 °C (105 °F).

There is also some limited evidence that supports sponging or bathing children suffering from fever with tepid water. The use of any ventilation appliances like fans or air conditioning may also somewhat reduce the temperature and increase the comfort of the person. If somehow the temperature reaches an extremely high level of hyperpyrexia, aggressive cooling may be required. In general, it is advised to keep most people adequately hydrated. Whether or not fluid intake improves symptoms or curtails respiratory illnesses such as the common cold is not yet known.

Medications that help lower some fevers are called antipyretics. The antipyretic, ibuprofen has been shown to be quite effective in reducing fevers in children. This is more effective than acetaminophen in children. Ibuprofen and acetaminophen can be safely used together in children with fevers. The effectiveness of acetaminophen by itself in children with fevers has been look into. Ibuprofen is also superior to aspirin in children with fever.

However, using aspirin is not recommended in children and young adults due to the higher risk of developing Reye's syndrome. Using paracetamol and ibuprofen at the same time or alternating among the two is more effective at decreasing fever than using only paracetamol or ibuprofen. It is unclear if it increases child comfort.

Other measures like putting a damp cloth on the forehead and having a slight warm bath may also help. Today, there are a lot of cooling pads that you can buy in stores that you can use to ease the fever. Children who are younger than three months with a fever should be medically assessed.

CONCLUSION

Keep in mind that not all treatments listed for each ailment is guaranteed to work 100 percent. These treatments are considered to be preventive measures that can help improve the condition of the one who happens to be suffering from that certain ailment. While it there may not be any full proof cures for most of these ailments, it is still strongly recommended for anyone to consult a doctor in the event when you or any of your family members contact any of these.

ALWAYS consult a doctor or your health practitioner on what

medications you should take to avoid any future problems and otherwise any negative side effects before taking drugs.